THIS JOURNAL BELONGS TO

_____

CREATED BY ARIELLE HAUGHEE

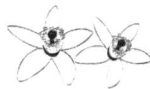

ORANGE BLOSSOM
PUBLISHING

MAITLAND, FLORIDA

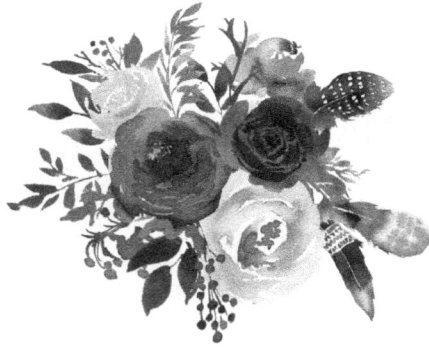

Published 2020 by Orange Blossom Publishing
Maitland, Florida
www.orangeblossombooks.com

ISBN: 978-1-949935-16-5

a Note from Arielle

You work hard. Incredibly hard. I know this because I used to be a teacher as well (ESE, 4th, 5th). You spend countless hours and way too many dollars making things work. You love all your kids dearly and give everything you have to help them succeed.

But there's someone else who needs attention, too: You.

Teaching is a profession that never seems to end; there is always more to do. You can easily sacrifice all of yourself in this career. In order to be the best teacher, the best person you can be, you need to find balance.

Take care of yourself, not just for your students, but because you deserve to have all the happiness life has to offer. Happy journaling!

MY GOALS FOR MYSELF

Sleep: ....

Exercise: ....

Food choices: ....
....

Family time:..

I will not work on this/these day(s):
....

I will not work past this time:
....

I will find strength by:
....
....
....
....

I will release stress by:
....
....
....
....

**I will fill out this journal on (day)................................at
(time)........................... .**

Student Name: Positive Trait:

....

....

....

....

....

....

....

....

....

....

....

....

....

....

....

....

....

....

....

....

....

Student Name: Positive Trait:

....

....

....

....

....

....

....

....

....

....

....

....

....

....

....

....

....

....

....

....

Student Name: Positive Trait:

....

....

....

....

....

....

....

....

....

....

....

....

....

....

....

....

....

....

....

....

WEEK 1

I am proud of myself for:

I am grateful for:

Things that worked well:

What didn't work well:

Something I need to let go of:

A student that made me smile:

I made things easier for myself by:

_____
_____
_____
_____
_____
_____
_____
_____

Something I did for myself:

It's not my fault that...

Something new to try next week:

_____
_____
_____
_____
_____
_____
_____
_____
_____
_____

My focus next week:

_____
_____
_____
_____
_____
_____
_____

Stressors next week:

WEEK 2

I am proud of myself for:
_____
_____
_____
_____
_____
_____
_____
_____

I am grateful for:

Things that worked well:
_____
_____
_____
_____
_____
_____
_____

What didn't work well:

Something I need to let go of:

A student that made me smile:
_____
_____
_____
_____
_____
_____

I made things easier
for myself by:

_____
_____
_____
_____
_____
_____

Something I did for myself:

It's not my fault that...

Something new to try
next week:

_____
_____
_____
_____
_____
_____
_____
_____
_____
_____

My focus next week:

_____
_____
_____
_____
_____
_____

Stressors next week:

WEEK 3

I am grateful for:

I am proud of myself for:

Things that worked well:

What didn't work well:

Something I need to let go of:

A student that made me smile:

I made things easier
for myself by:
_____
_____
_____
_____
_____
_____
_____

Something I did for myself:

It's not my fault that...

Something new to try
next week:
_____
_____
_____
_____
_____
_____
_____
_____
_____

My focus next week:
_____
_____
_____
_____
_____
_____

Stressors next week:

WEEK 4

I am proud of myself for:

I am grateful for:

Things that worked well:

What didn't work well:

Something I need to let go of:

A student that made me smile:

I made things easier
for myself by:

_____

_____

_____

_____

_____

_____

_____

Something I did for myself:

It's not my fault that...

Something new to try
next week:

_____

_____

_____

_____

_____

_____

_____

_____

My focus next week:

_____

_____

_____

_____

_____

_____

Stressors next week:

Give some of the love you give to the kids to yourself.

POSITIVE THINGS PEOPLE SAY ABOUT ME

My students: ....

....

....

My classroom parents: ....

....

....

My peers: ....

....

....

My family: ....

....

....

Other: ....

....

GOAL CHECK IN:

Look back at your goals from the beginning of this journal.

Are you meeting your sleep goal?

Are you meeting your exercise goal?

Are you meeting your food choices goal?

Are you meeting your family time goal?

Are you not working on the day/days you said you wouldn't?

Are you not working past the time you said you wouldn't?

WEEK 5

I am proud of myself for:

I am grateful for:

Things that worked well:

What didn't work well:

Something I need to let go of:

A student that made me smile:

I made things easier
for myself by:

_____
_____
_____
_____
_____
_____
_____

Something I did for myself:

It's not my fault that...

Something new to try
next week:

_____
_____
_____
_____
_____
_____
_____
_____

My focus next week:

_____
_____
_____
_____
_____
_____
_____

Stressors next week:

WEEK 6

I am proud of myself for:

I am grateful for:

Things that worked well:

What didn't work well:

Something I need to let go of:

A student that made me smile:

I made things easier for myself by:

_____
_____
_____
_____
_____
_____
_____

Something I did for myself:

It's not my fault that...

Something new to try next week:

_____
_____
_____
_____
_____
_____
_____
_____

My focus next week:

_____
_____
_____
_____
_____
_____

Stressors next week:

WEEK 7

I am grateful for:

I am proud of myself for:

Things that worked well:

What didn't work well:

Something I need to let go of:

A student that made me smile:

I made things easier
for myself by:

_____
_____
_____
_____
_____
_____
_____

Something I did for myself:

It's not my fault that...

Something new to try
next week:

_____
_____
_____
_____
_____
_____
_____
_____
_____

My focus next week:

_____
_____
_____
_____
_____
_____
_____

Stressors next week:

WEEK 8

I am proud of myself for:

I am grateful for:

Things that worked well:

What didn't work well:

Something I need to let go of:

A student that made me smile:

I made things easier
for myself by:
_____
_____
_____
_____
_____
_____
_____

Something I did for myself:

It's not my fault that...

Something new to try
next week:
_____
_____
_____
_____
_____
_____
_____

My focus next week:
_____
_____
_____
_____
_____
_____

Stressors next week:

Remember YOU are worth your time, too.

RECOGNIZING AND ADJUSTING THOUGHT PATTERNS

Things that make me feel overwhelmed: ....
....
....

Positive phrase to tell myself so I can move forward:
....
....

Things that make me feel like a failure: ....
....
....

Positive phrase to tell myself so I can move forward:
....
....

Activities to help me reset when having a bad day:
....

GOAL CHECK IN:

Look back at your goals from the beginning of this journal.

Are you meeting your sleep goal?
Are you meeting your exercise goal?
Are you meeting your food choices goal?
Are you meeting your family time goal?
Are you not working on the day/days you said you wouldn't?
Are you not working past the time you said you wouldn't?

WEEK 9

I am grateful for:

I am proud of myself for:

Things that worked well:

What didn't work well:

Something I need to let go of:

A student that made me smile:

I made things easier
for myself by:

_____

_____

_____

_____

_____

_____

Something I did for myself:

It's not my fault that...

Something new to try
next week:

_____

_____

_____

_____

_____

_____

_____

_____

My focus next week:

_____

_____

_____

_____

_____

_____

Stressors next week:

WEEK 10

I am grateful for:

I am proud of myself for:

Things that worked well:

What didn't work well:

Something I need to let go of:

A student that made me smile:

I made things easier
for myself by:

_____
_____
_____
_____
_____
_____
_____

Something I did for myself:

It's not my fault that...

Something new to try
next week:

_____
_____
_____
_____
_____
_____
_____
_____

My focus next week:

_____
_____
_____
_____
_____
_____
_____

Stressors next week:

WEEK 11

I am grateful for:

I am proud of myself for:
_____
_____
_____
_____
_____
_____
_____
_____
_____

Things that worked well:
_____
_____
_____
_____
_____
_____

What didn't work well:

Something I need to let go of:

A student that made me smile:
_____
_____
_____
_____
_____
_____

I made things easier for myself by:

Something I did for myself:

It's not my fault that...

Something new to try next week:

My focus next week:

Stressors next week:

WEEK 12

I am proud of myself for:

I am grateful for:

Things that worked well:

What didn't work well:

Something I need to let go of:

A student that made me smile:

I made things easier for myself by:

_____
_____
_____
_____
_____
_____
_____

Something I did for myself:

It's not my fault that...

Something new to try next week:

_____
_____
_____
_____
_____
_____
_____
_____
_____

My focus next week:

_____
_____
_____
_____
_____
_____
_____

Stressors next week:

You perform little miracles every single day.

PEOPLE WHO INSPIRE OR ENERGIZE ME

Plan to spend more time with those who are uplifting.

Family members: ....

....

....

Friends: ....

....

....

Colleagues: ....

....

....

Ideas for meeting new uplifting people: ....

....

....

GOAL CHECK IN:

Look back at your goals from the beginning of this journal.

Are you meeting your sleep goal?

Are you meeting your exercise goal?

Are you meeting your food choices goal?

Are you meeting your family time goal?

Are you not working on the day/days you said you wouldn't?

Are you not working past the time you said you wouldn't?

WEEK 13

I am proud of myself for:

I am grateful for:

Things that worked well:

What didn't work well:

Something I need to let go of:

A student that made me smile:

I made things easier for myself by:

_____
_____
_____
_____
_____
_____
_____

Something I did for myself:

It's not my fault that...

Something new to try next week:

_____
_____
_____
_____
_____
_____
_____
_____

My focus next week:

_____
_____
_____
_____
_____
_____
_____

Stressors next week:

WEEK 14

I am proud of myself for:
_____
_____
_____
_____
_____
_____
_____
_____

I am grateful for:

Things that worked well:
_____
_____
_____
_____
_____
_____
_____

What didn't work well:

Something I need to let go of:

A student that made me smile:
_____
_____
_____
_____
_____
_____

I made things easier
for myself by:

_____
_____
_____
_____
_____
_____
_____

Something I did for myself:

It's not my fault that...

Something new to try
next week:
_____
_____
_____
_____
_____
_____
_____
_____
_____
_____

My focus next week:
_____
_____
_____
_____
_____
_____
_____

Stressors next week:

WEEK 15

I am proud of myself for:

I am grateful for:

Things that worked well:

What didn't work well:

Something I need to let go of:

A student that made me smile:

I made things easier
for myself by:
_____

Something I did for myself:

It's not my fault that...

Something new to try
next week:
_____

My focus next week:
_____

Stressors next week:

WEEK 16

I am proud of myself for:

I am grateful for:

Things that worked well:

What didn't work well:

Something I need to let go of:

A student that made me smile:

I made things easier for myself by:

Something I did for myself:

It's not my fault that...

Something new to try next week:

My focus next week:

Stressors next week:

Create an
environment of
acceptance, starting
with yourself.

SOMETHING I WANT TO FORGET

Write the memory on this page. Any time it pops in your head, tell yourself those words are here on this paper and nowhere else. Then refocus.

....

....

....

....

....

....

....

....

....

....

....

....

GOAL CHECK IN:

Look back at your goals from the beginning of this journal.

Are you meeting your sleep goal?
Are you meeting your exercise goal?
Are you meeting your food choices goal?
Are you meeting your family time goal?
Are you not working on the day/days you said you wouldn't?
Are you not working past the time you said you wouldn't?

WEEK 17

I am proud of myself for:

I am grateful for:

Things that worked well:

What didn't work well:

Something I need to let go of:

A student that made me smile:

I made things easier
for myself by:
_____
_____
_____
_____
_____
_____
_____

Something I did for myself:

It's not my fault that...

Something new to try
next week:
_____
_____
_____
_____
_____
_____
_____
_____

My focus next week:
_____
_____
_____
_____
_____
_____
_____

Stressors next week:

WEEK 18

I am proud of myself for:

I am grateful for:

Things that worked well:

What didn't work well:

Something I need to let go of:

A student that made me smile:

I made things easier
for myself by:

_____

_____

_____

_____

_____

_____

Something I did for myself:

It's not my fault that...

Something new to try
next week:

_____

_____

_____

_____

_____

_____

_____

_____

My focus next week:

_____

_____

_____

_____

_____

_____

Stressors next week:

WEEK 19

I am grateful for:

I am proud of myself for:

Things that worked well:

What didn't work well:

Something I need to let go of:

A student that made me smile:

I made things easier for myself by:

_____

_____

_____

_____

_____

_____

_____

Something I did for myself:

It's not my fault that...

Something new to try next week:

_____

_____

_____

_____

_____

_____

_____

_____

My focus next week:

_____

_____

_____

_____

_____

_____

Stressors next week:

WEEK 20

I am proud of myself for:

I am grateful for:

Things that worked well:

What didn't work well:

Something I need to let go of:

A student that made me smile:

I made things easier for myself by:

_____

_____

_____

_____

_____

_____

_____

Something I did for myself:

It's not my fault that...

Something new to try next week:

_____

_____

_____

_____

_____

_____

_____

_____

_____

My focus next week:

_____

_____

_____

_____

_____

_____

Stressors next week:

Choose happiness.

HOME AREAS TO FOCUS ON

Cleaning, organizing, or sprucing up different areas in your home can have a big impact on your happiness. Set goals for completing areas.

Living areas: ....
....

Bedrooms: ....
....

Bathrooms: ....
....

Kitchen: ....
....

Dining room: ....
....

Garage: ....
....

Other: ....

GOAL CHECK IN:

Look back at your goals from the beginning of this journal.

Are you meeting your sleep goal?
Are you meeting your exercise goal?
Are you meeting your food choices goal?
Are you meeting your family time goal?
Are you not working on the day/days you said you wouldn't?
Are you not working past the time you said you wouldn't?

WEEK 21

I am proud of myself for:

I am grateful for:

Things that worked well:

What didn't work well:

Something I need to let go of:

A student that made me smile:

I made things easier for myself by:

_____
_____
_____
_____
_____
_____
_____
_____

Something I did for myself:

It's not my fault that...

Something new to try next week:

_____
_____
_____
_____
_____
_____
_____
_____
_____

My focus next week:

_____
_____
_____
_____
_____
_____

Stressors next week:

WEEK 22

I am proud of myself for:
_____
_____
_____
_____
_____
_____
_____
_____

I am grateful for:

Things that worked well:
_____
_____
_____
_____
_____
_____

What didn't work well:

Something I need to let go of:

A student that made
me smile:
_____
_____
_____
_____
_____

I made things easier
for myself by:
_____
_____
_____
_____
_____
_____
_____

Something I did for myself:

It's not my fault that...

Something new to try
next week:
_____
_____
_____
_____
_____
_____
_____
_____
_____

My focus next week:
_____
_____
_____
_____
_____
_____

Stressors next week:

WEEK 23

I am grateful for:

I am proud of myself for:

Things that worked well:

What didn't work well:

Something I need to let go of:

A student that made me smile:

I made things easier
for myself by:

_____
_____
_____
_____
_____
_____
_____

Something I did for myself:

It's not my fault that...

Something new to try
next week:

_____
_____
_____
_____
_____
_____
_____
_____
_____

My focus next week:

_____
_____
_____
_____
_____
_____

Stressors next week:

WEEK 24

I am grateful for:

I am proud of myself for:

Things that worked well:

What didn't work well:

Something I need to let go of:

A student that made me smile:

I made things easier
for myself by:

_____
_____
_____
_____
_____
_____
_____

Something I did for myself:

It's not my fault that...

Something new to try
next week:

_____
_____
_____
_____
_____
_____
_____
_____
_____

My focus next week:

_____
_____
_____
_____
_____
_____
_____

Stressors next week:

You are shaping the future for us all.

WAYS TO ENJOY NATURE

Think of places you can walk or perhaps drive to where you can enjoy the outdoors. Make a plan to visit some of these places this month.

....

....

....

....

....

....

....

....

....

....

....

....

....

GOAL CHECK IN:

Look back at your goals from the beginning of this journal.

Are you meeting your sleep goal?
Are you meeting your exercise goal?
Are you meeting your food choices goal?
Are you meeting your family time goal?
Are you not working on the day/days you said you wouldn't?
Are you not working past the time you said you wouldn't?

WEEK 25

I am proud of myself for:
_____
_____
_____
_____
_____
_____
_____

I am grateful for:

Things that worked well:
_____
_____
_____
_____
_____

What didn't work well:

Something I need to let go of:

A student that made me smile:
_____
_____
_____
_____

I made things easier
for myself by:
_____
_____
_____
_____
_____
_____
_____

Something I did for myself:

It's not my fault that...

Something new to try
next week:
_____
_____
_____
_____
_____
_____
_____
_____
_____

My focus next week:
_____
_____
_____
_____
_____
_____
_____

Stressors next week:

WEEK 26

I am grateful for:

I am proud of myself for:

Things that worked well:

What didn't work well:

Something I need to let go of:

A student that made me smile:

I made things easier
for myself by:

_____
_____
_____
_____
_____
_____
_____

Something I did for myself:

It's not my fault that...

Something new to try
next week:

_____
_____
_____
_____
_____
_____
_____
_____
_____

My focus next week:

_____
_____
_____
_____
_____
_____

Stressors next week:

WEEK 27

I am proud of myself for:

I am grateful for:

Things that worked well:

What didn't work well:

Something I need to let go of:

A student that made me smile:

I made things easier for myself by:

_____
_____
_____
_____
_____
_____
_____
_____

Something I did for myself:

It's not my fault that...

Something new to try next week:

_____
_____
_____
_____
_____
_____
_____
_____
_____

My focus next week:

_____
_____
_____
_____
_____
_____
_____

Stressors next week:

WEEK 28

I am proud of myself for:
_____
_____
_____
_____
_____
_____
_____

I am grateful for:

Things that worked well:
_____
_____
_____
_____
_____
_____

What didn't work well:

Something I need to let go of:

A student that made me smile:
_____
_____
_____
_____
_____
_____

I made things easier
for myself by:

_____
_____
_____
_____
_____
_____
_____

Something I did for myself:

It's not my fault that...

Something new to try
next week:

_____
_____
_____
_____
_____
_____
_____
_____
_____

My focus next week:

_____
_____
_____
_____
_____
_____
_____

Stressors next week:

Teach patience by being patient with yourself.

SLEEP DIARY

Monday
Hours Slept: ....
Notes: ....

Tuesday
Hours Slept: ....
Notes: ....

Wednesday
Hours Slept: ....
Notes: ....

Thursday
Hours Slept: ....
Notes: ....

Friday
Hours Slept: ....
Notes: ....

Weekend
Hours Slept: ....
Notes: ....

GOAL CHECK IN:

Look back at your goals from the beginning of this journal.

Are you meeting your sleep goal?
Are you meeting your exercise goal?
Are you meeting your food choices goal?
Are you meeting your family time goal?
Are you not working on the day/days you said you wouldn't?
Are you not working past the time you said you wouldn't?

WEEK 29

I am grateful for:

I am proud of myself for:

Things that worked well:

What didn't work well:

Something I need to let go of:

A student that made me smile:

I made things easier
for myself by:
_____
_____
_____
_____
_____
_____
_____
_____

Something I did for myself:

It's not my fault that...

Something new to try
next week:
_____
_____
_____
_____
_____
_____
_____
_____
_____

My focus next week:
_____
_____
_____
_____
_____
_____
_____

Stressors next week:

WEEK 30

I am proud of myself for:

I am grateful for:

Things that worked well:

What didn't work well:

Something I need to let go of:

A student that made me smile:

I made things easier
for myself by:
_____
_____
_____
_____
_____
_____
_____

Something I did for myself:

It's not my fault that...

Something new to try
next week:
_____
_____
_____
_____
_____
_____
_____
_____
_____
_____

My focus next week:
_____
_____
_____
_____
_____
_____
_____

Stressors next week:

WEEK 31

I am proud of myself for:

I am grateful for:

Things that worked well:

What didn't work well:

Something I need to let go of:

A student that made me smile:

I made things easier
for myself by:
_____
_____
_____
_____
_____
_____

Something I did for myself:

It's not my fault that...

Something new to try
next week:
_____
_____
_____
_____
_____
_____
_____
_____
_____

My focus next week:
_____
_____
_____
_____
_____
_____
_____

Stressors next week:

WEEK 32

I am grateful for:

I am proud of myself for:

Things that worked well:

What didn't work well:

Something I need to let go of:

A student that made me smile:

I made things easier
for myself by:

_____
_____
_____
_____
_____
_____

Something I did for myself:

It's not my fault that...

Something new to try
next week:

_____
_____
_____
_____
_____
_____
_____
_____

My focus next week:

_____
_____
_____
_____
_____
_____

Stressors next week:

Living a balanced
life allows you to be
a better teacher.

A MEMORY I WANT TO KEEP FOREVER

....
....
....
....
....
....
....
....
....
....
....
....
....
....

GOAL CHECK IN:

Look back at your goals from the beginning of this journal.

Are you meeting your sleep goal?

Are you meeting your exercise goal?

Are you meeting your food choices goal?

Are you meeting your family time goal?

Are you not working on the day/days you said you wouldn't?

Are you not working past the time you said you wouldn't?

WEEK 33

I am proud of myself for:

I am grateful for:

Things that worked well:

What didn't work well:

Something I need to let go of:

A student that made me smile:

I made things easier
for myself by:
_____
_____
_____
_____
_____
_____
_____

Something I did for myself:

It's not my fault that...

Something new to try
next week:
_____
_____
_____
_____
_____
_____
_____
_____
_____
_____

My focus next week:
_____
_____
_____
_____
_____
_____
_____

Stressors next week:

WEEK 34

I am grateful for:

I am proud of myself for:

Things that worked well:

What didn't work well:

Something I need to let go of:

A student that made me smile:

I made things easier for myself by:

_____
_____
_____
_____
_____
_____

Something I did for myself:

It's not my fault that...

Something new to try next week:

_____
_____
_____
_____
_____
_____
_____
_____

My focus next week:

_____
_____
_____
_____
_____
_____

Stressors next week:

WEEK 35

I am proud of myself for:

I am grateful for:

Things that worked well:

What didn't work well:

Something I need to let go of:

A student that made me smile:

I made things easier
for myself by:
_____
_____
_____
_____
_____
_____
_____
_____

Something I did for myself:

It's not my fault that...

Something new to try
next week:
_____
_____
_____
_____
_____
_____
_____
_____
_____
_____

My focus next week:
_____
_____
_____
_____
_____
_____
_____

Stressors next week:

WEEK 36

I am grateful for:

I am proud of myself for:

Things that worked well:

What didn't work well:

Something I need to let go of:

A student that made me smile:

I made things easier
for myself by:
_____
_____
_____
_____
_____
_____

Something I did for myself:

It's not my fault that...

Something new to try
next week:
_____
_____
_____
_____
_____
_____
_____
_____
_____

My focus next week:
_____
_____
_____
_____
_____
_____

Stressors next week:

Allow yourself to laugh with the kids and have fun.

EVALUATE HOW YOU DEFINE SUCCESS

What does success mean to you? ....
....
....
....
....

How do different elements of your life (teaching, family, wellness...) fit into your definition?
....
....
....
....

When will you celebrate your success?
....
....
....

GOAL CHECK IN:

Look back at your goals from the beginning of this journal.

Are you meeting your sleep goal?
Are you meeting your exercise goal?
Are you meeting your food choices goal?
Are you meeting your family time goal?
Are you not working on the day/days you said you wouldn't?
Are you not working past the time you said you wouldn't?

WEEK 37

I am grateful for:

I am proud of myself for:

Things that worked well:

What didn't work well:

Something I need to let go of:

A student that made me smile:

I made things easier
for myself by:
_____
_____
_____
_____
_____
_____
_____

Something I did for myself:

It's not my fault that...

Something new to try
next week:
_____
_____
_____
_____
_____
_____
_____
_____
_____

My focus next week:
_____
_____
_____
_____
_____
_____

Stressors next week:

WEEK 38

I am grateful for:

I am proud of myself for:

Things that worked well:

What didn't work well:

Something I need to let go of:

A student that made me smile:

I made things easier
for myself by:

Something I did for myself:

It's not my fault that...

Something new to try
next week:

My focus next week:

Stressors next week:

WEEK 39

I am proud of myself for:
_____
_____
_____
_____
_____
_____
_____
_____

I am grateful for:

Things that worked well:
_____
_____
_____
_____
_____

What didn't work well:

Something I need to let go of:

A student that made me smile:
_____
_____
_____
_____
_____
_____

I made things easier
for myself by:

_____
_____
_____
_____
_____
_____
_____
_____

Something I did for myself:

It's not my fault that...

Something new to try
next week:

_____
_____
_____
_____
_____
_____
_____
_____
_____
_____

My focus next week:

_____
_____
_____
_____
_____
_____
_____

Stressors next week:

WEEK 40

I am proud of myself for:

I am grateful for:

Things that worked well:

What didn't work well:

Something I need to let go of:

A student that made me smile:

I made things easier for myself by:

_____
_____
_____
_____
_____
_____

Something I did for myself:

It's not my fault that...

Something new to try next week:

_____
_____
_____
_____
_____
_____
_____
_____
_____

My focus next week:

_____
_____
_____
_____
_____
_____

Stressors next week:

Some parents are just plain crazy. It's not you!

IDEAS FOR INCORPORATING MORE EXERCISE

....

....

....

....

....

....

....

....

....

....

....

....

....

....

GOAL CHECK IN:

Look back at your goals from the beginning of this journal.

Are you meeting your sleep goal?
Are you meeting your exercise goal?
Are you meeting your food choices goal?
Are you meeting your family time goal?
Are you not working on the day/days you said you wouldn't?
Are you not working past the time you said you wouldn't?

WEEK 41

I am grateful for:

I am proud of myself for:

Things that worked well:

What didn't work well:

Something I need to let go of:

A student that made me smile:

I made things easier
for myself by:

_____
_____
_____
_____
_____
_____
_____

Something I did for myself:

It's not my fault that...

Something new to try
next week:

_____
_____
_____
_____
_____
_____
_____
_____
_____

My focus next week:

_____
_____
_____
_____
_____
_____
_____

Stressors next week:

WEEK 42

I am grateful for:

I am proud of myself for:

Things that worked well:

What didn't work well:

Something I need to let go of:

A student that made me smile:

I made things easier
for myself by: _____
_____
_____
_____
_____
_____
_____
_____

Something I did for myself:

It's not my fault that...

Something new to try
next week:
_____
_____
_____
_____
_____
_____
_____
_____
_____
_____
_____

My focus next week:
_____
_____
_____
_____
_____
_____
_____

Stressors next week:

WEEK 43

I am grateful for:

I am proud of myself for:

Things that worked well:

What didn't work well:

Something I need to let go of:

A student that made me smile:

I made things easier
for myself by:
_____
_____
_____
_____
_____
_____
_____

Something I did for myself:

It's not my fault that...

Something new to try
next week:
_____
_____
_____
_____
_____
_____
_____
_____
_____
_____

My focus next week:
_____
_____
_____
_____
_____
_____
_____

Stressors next week:

WEEK 44

I am grateful for:

I am proud of myself for:

Things that worked well:

What didn't work well:

Something I need to let go of:

A student that made me smile:

I made things easier for myself by:

_____
_____
_____
_____
_____
_____

Something I did for myself:

It's not my fault that...

Something new to try next week:

_____
_____
_____
_____
_____
_____
_____
_____

My focus next week:

_____
_____
_____
_____
_____
_____

Stressors next week:

Don't lose yourself while you are trying to be everything to your kids.

RECONNECT WITH YOUR WHY

Why did you decide to become a teacher? ....

....

....

Why do you put forth so much time and effort?: ....

....

....

Why is your job important in society? ....

....

....

Why do you love teaching?: ....

....

....

Why are you doing this journal?: ....

....

GOAL CHECK IN:

Look back at your goals from the beginning of this journal.

Are you meeting your sleep goal?
Are you meeting your exercise goal?
Are you meeting your food choices goal?
Are you meeting your family time goal?
Are you not working on the day/days you said you wouldn't?
Are you not working past the time you said you wouldn't?

WEEK 45

I am proud of myself for:

I am grateful for:

Things that worked well:

What didn't work well:

Something I need to let go of:

A student that made me smile:

I made things easier
for myself by:

_____
_____
_____
_____
_____
_____
_____

Something I did for myself:

It's not my fault that...

Something new to try
next week:

_____
_____
_____
_____
_____
_____
_____
_____
_____
_____

My focus next week:

_____
_____
_____
_____
_____
_____
_____

Stressors next week:

WEEK 46

I am grateful for:

I am proud of myself for:

Things that worked well:

What didn't work well:

Something I need to let go of:

A student that made me smile:

I made things easier
for myself by:

_____
_____
_____
_____
_____
_____
_____

Something I did for myself:

It's not my fault that...

Something new to try
next week:

_____
_____
_____
_____
_____
_____
_____
_____

My focus next week:

_____
_____
_____
_____
_____
_____

Stressors next week:

WEEK 47

I am proud of myself for:

I am grateful for:

Things that worked well:

What didn't work well:

Something I need to let go of:

A student that made me smile:

I made things easier for myself by:

_____

_____

_____

_____

_____

_____

Something I did for myself:

It's not my fault that...

Something new to try next week:

_____

_____

_____

_____

_____

_____

_____

_____

My focus next week:

_____

_____

_____

_____

_____

_____

Stressors next week:

WEEK 48

I am grateful for:

I am proud of myself for:

Things that worked well:

What didn't work well:

Something I need to let go of:

A student that made me smile:

I made things easier
for myself by:
_____
_____
_____
_____
_____
_____
_____

Something I did for myself:

It's not my fault that...

Something new to try
next week:
_____
_____
_____
_____
_____
_____
_____
_____
_____

My focus next week:
_____
_____
_____
_____
_____
_____
_____

Stressors next week:

Your classroom is
a world that you
create.

NEGATIVE PEOPLE I NEED TO LIMIT TIME WITH

We can't always control who is in our lives, but we can try and control how much we interact with them.

Family members: ....
....
....

Friends: ....
....
....

Colleagues: ....
....
....

Ideas for a quick escape: ....
....
....

GOAL CHECK IN:

Look back at your goals from the beginning of this journal.

Are you meeting your sleep goal?
Are you meeting your exercise goal?
Are you meeting your food choices goal?
Are you meeting your family time goal?
Are you not working on the day/days you said you wouldn't?
Are you not working past the time you said you wouldn't?

WEEK 49

I am grateful for:

I am proud of myself for:

Things that worked well:

What didn't work well:

Something I need to let go of:

A student that made me smile:

I made things easier
for myself by:

_____

_____

_____

_____

_____

_____

_____

Something I did for myself:

It's not my fault that...

Something new to try
next week:

_____

_____

_____

_____

_____

_____

_____

_____

My focus next week:

_____

_____

_____

_____

_____

_____

Stressors next week:

WEEK 50

I am proud of myself for:

I am grateful for:

Things that worked well:

What didn't work well:

Something I need to let go of:

A student that made me smile:

I made things easier
for myself by:

_____
_____
_____
_____
_____
_____
_____

Something I did for myself:

It's not my fault that...

Something new to try
next week:

_____
_____
_____
_____
_____
_____
_____
_____
_____
_____

My focus next week:

_____
_____
_____
_____
_____
_____
_____

Stressors next week:

WEEK 51

I am proud of myself for:

I am grateful for:

Things that worked well:

What didn't work well:

Something I need to let go of:

A student that made me smile:

I made things easier
for myself by:

_____
_____
_____
_____
_____
_____
_____

Something I did for myself:

It's not my fault that...

Something new to try
next week:

_____
_____
_____
_____
_____
_____
_____
_____
_____

My focus next week:

_____
_____
_____
_____
_____
_____

Stressors next week:

WEEK 52

I am proud of myself for:

I am grateful for:

Things that worked well:

What didn't work well:

Something I need to let go of:

A student that made me smile:

I made things easier for myself by:

_____
_____
_____
_____
_____
_____

Something I did for myself:

It's not my fault that...

Something new to try next week:

_____
_____
_____
_____
_____
_____
_____
_____

My focus next week:

_____
_____
_____
_____
_____
_____

Stressors next week:

END OF YEAR REFLECTION

High point of the year: ....

....

....

....

....

Low point of the year: ....

....

....

....

I am most proud of: ....

....

....

....

How I feel I maintained balance: ....

....

....

....

Things I want to try next year: ....

....

....

....

NOTES

....
....
....
....
....
....
....
....
....
....
....
....
....
....
....
....
....
....
....
....
....
....

Other Journals from Orange Blossom

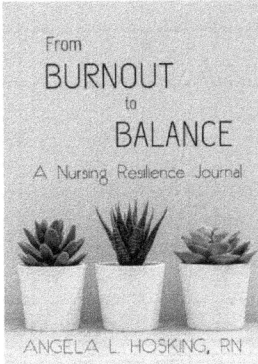

From Burnout to Balance:
A Nursing Resilience Journal

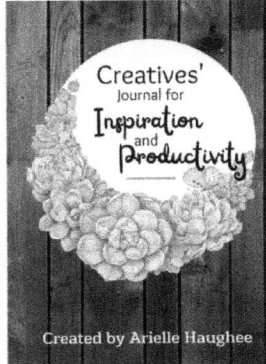

Creatives' Journal for
Inspiration and Productivity

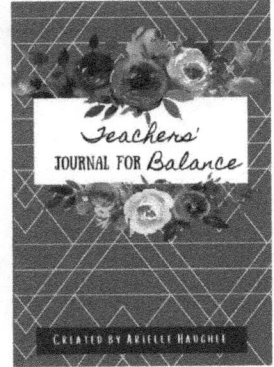

Teachers' Journal for
Balance

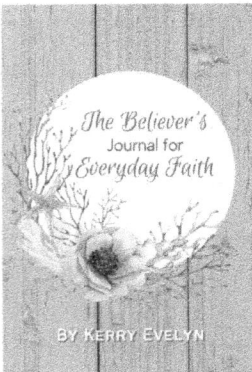

The Believer's Journal for
Everyday Faith

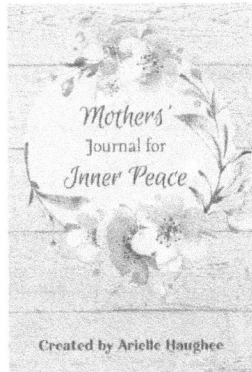

Mothers' Journal for
Inner Peace

Scan here to see the
journals and other
great books!

www.ingramcontent.com/pod-product-compliance
Lightning Source LLC
Chambersburg PA
CBHW022059020426
42335CB00012B/756